The Sirtfood Diet Recipe Book

50 Easy and Delicious Recipes to Activate Sirtuins. The Cookbook to Lose Weight Get Lean and Feel Great! Burn Fat and Stay Fit.

Kate Matten

Table of Contents

4

Explanation of Sirt Food Diet

What is The Sirtfood Diet?

Launched originally in 2016, the Sirtfood diet remains a hot topic and involves followers adopting a diet rich in 'sirtfoods'. According to the diet's founders, these special foods work by activating specific proteins in the body called sirtuins. Sirtuins are believed to protect cells in the body from dying when they are under stress and are thought to regulate inflammation, metabolism, and the aging process. It's thought that sirtuins influence the body's ability to burn fat and boost metabolism, resulting in a seven-pound weight loss a week while maintaining muscle. However, some experts believe this is unlikely to be solely fat loss, but will instead reflect changes in glycogen stores from skeletal muscle and the liver.

So What Are These Magical 'Sirtfoods'? The Twenty Most Common Include:

- ❖ kale
- ❖ red wine
- ❖ strawberries
- ❖ onions
- ❖ soy

- parsley
- extra virgin olive oil
- dark chocolate (85% cocoa)
- matcha green tea
- buckwheat
- turmeric
- walnuts
- arugula (rocket)
- bird's eye chili
- lovage
- Medjool dates
- red chicory
- blueberries
- capers
- coffee

The diet is divided into two phases; the initial phase lasts one week and involves restricting calories to 1000kcal for three days, consuming three sirtfood green juices, and one meal rich in sirtfoods each day. The juices include kale, celery, rocket, parsley, green tea, and lemon. Meals include turkey escalope with sage, capers and parsley, chicken and kale curry, and prawn stir-fry with buckwheat noodles. From days four to seven, energy intakes are increased to 1500kcal comprising of two sirtfood green juices and two sirtfood-rich meals a day. Although the diet promotes healthy foods, it's restrictive in both your food choices and daily calories, especially during the initial stages. It also involves drinking juice, with the amounts suggested during phase one exceeding the current daily guidelines.

The second phase is known as the maintenance phase which lasts 14 days where steady weight loss occurs. The authors believe it's a sustainable and realistic way to lose weight. However, focusing on weight loss is not what the diet is all about – it's designed to be about eating the best foods nature has to offer. Long term they recommend eating three balanced sirtfood rich meals a day along with one sirtfood green juice.

Dietitian Emer Delaney Says:

'At first glance, this is not a diet I would advise for my clients. Aiming to have 1000kcal for three consecutive days is extremely difficult and I believe the majority of people would be unable to achieve it. Looking at the list of foods, you can see they are the sort of items that often appear on a 'healthy food list', however it would be better to encourage these as part of a healthy balanced diet. Having a glass of red wine or a small amount of chocolate occasionally won't do us any harm – I wouldn't recommend them daily. We should also be eating a mixture of different fruits and vegetables and not just those on the list.

There are 20 SIRT1 activating foods you can include in your diet to lose weight, get rid of stubborn belly fat, and restore muscle mass. Take a look at the table below:

Sirtfoods

	Sirtuin-Activating Foods	Nutrients
1	Arugula	Quercetin, kaempferol
2	Buckwheat	Rutin
3	Capers	Kaempferol, quercetin
4	Celery (with leaves)	Apigenin, luteolin
5	Chilies	Luteolin, myricetin
6	Cocoa	Epicatechin
7	Coffee	Caffeic acid
8	Extra virgin olive oil	Oleuropein, hydroxytyrosol

9	Garlic	Ajoene, myricetin
10	Green tea (especially matcha)	Epigallocatechin gallate (EGCG)
11	Kale Kaempferol,	Quercetin
12	Medjool dates	Gallic acid, caffeic acid
13	Parsley	Apigenin, myricetin
14	Red endive	Luteolin
15	Red onion	Quercetin
16	Red wine	Resveratrol, piceatannol
17	Soy	Daidzein, formononetin
18	Strawberries	Setin
19	Turmeric	Curcumin
20	Walnuts	Gallic acid

You can also include fish, chicken, and beef as they also are sirtuin-activating foods. These 20, however, should be the main focus on the plate.

40 Other Sirtfoods

You will now be familiar with the top 20 Sirtfoods and it is recommended that these foods retain a prominent part of your daily eating routine. This will ensure continued weight loss and overall well-being. There are, however, an additional 40 foods that also have Sirtfood properties. As variety is the spice of life you are actively encouraged to include these foods to expand the range of your diet.

In The Vegetable Category, These Foods Have Significant Sirtuin-Activating Nutrients.

- ❖ Artichokes
- ❖ Asparagus
- ❖ Bok choy/pak choi
- ❖ Broccoli
- ❖ Endive
- ❖ Green beans
- ❖ Shallots
- ❖ Watercress
- ❖ White onions
- ❖ Yellow chicory

In the Fruits category, these have significant sirtuin-activating nutrients

Apples

- ❖ Black plums
- ❖ Blackberries
- ❖ Blackcurrants
- ❖ Cranberries
- ❖ Goji berries
- ❖ Kumquats
- ❖ Raspberries
- ❖ Red grapes

In The Nuts And Seeds Category, These Have Significant Sirtuin-Activating Nutrients

- ❖ Chestnuts
- ❖ Chia seeds
- ❖ Peanuts
- ❖ Pecan nuts
- ❖ Pistachio nuts
- ❖ Sunflower seeds

In The Grains, Pseudo-Grains, And Beans Categories These Have Significant Sirtuin-Activating Nutrients

- ❖ Popcorn
- ❖ quinoa
- ❖ wholemeal flour
- ❖ broad beans
- ❖ white beans(e.g cannellini or haricot)

In The Herbs And Spices And Beverages. Categories These Have Significant Sirtuin-Activating Nutrients

- ❖ Chives
- ❖ Dill (fresh and dried)
- ❖ Dried oregano
- ❖ Dried sage
- ❖ Ginger
- ❖ Peppermint (fresh and dried)
- ❖ Standard chilies/hot peppers
- ❖ Thyme
- ❖ Black tea
- ❖ White tea
- ❖ Herbal tea

The diet combines sirt foods and calorie restriction, both of which may trigger the body to produce higher levels of sirtuins. The Sirtfood Diet book includes meal plans and recipes to follow, but there are plenty of other Sirtfood Diet recipe books available. The diet's creators claim that following the Sirtfood Diet will lead to rapid weight loss, all while maintaining muscle mass and protecting you from chronic disease. Once you have completed the diet, you're encouraged to continue including sirt foods and the diet's signature green juice into your regular diet.

With the Sirtfood diet, dieters can avoid severe calorie-restricted diets, have more energy, lose fat fast without losing muscle, and do not have to perform grueling exercise routines. The diet is certainly a relief from the other bland and demanding diet plans, like the GM diet. What happens when you are on the Sirtfood diet? Find out in the next section.

How Does The Sirtfood Diet Work? Is It Effective For Weight Loss?

The Sirtfood diet includes foods that activate SIRT1 genes. This diet is full of healthy foods that switch the

SIRT1 genes on and effectively trigger weight loss at the molecular level. Here's how the Sirtfood diet works:

1. Mobilizes The Fat: Scientists have found that the foods included in the Sirtfood diet help morph the stored white adipose tissue to brown fat, which gets readily mobilized and used up as energy. This means that the stored fat starts to melt and leads to weight loss.

2. Prevents Fat Accumulation: The SIRT1 genes regulate adipokine expression. Adipokines are secreted by fat cells that affect insulin sensitivity and hunger and increase inflammation. The SIRT1 gene activation through foods included in the Sirtfood diet helps reduce adipokine secretion. This prevents excessive fat accumulation and untimely hunger.

3. Improves Insulin Sensitivity: The inability of the cells to respond to insulin (a hormone responsible for uptake of glucose from the bloodstream by cells) leads to increased blood sugar levels, obesity, and Type 2 diabetes. Research shows that activating SIRT1 genes improves insulin sensitivity. This, in turn, improves metabolism, enhances the release of thyroid hormones, burns fatter, and protects against high-fat induced obesity.

4. Controls Excessive Hunger: Leptin is a hormone secreted by fat cells to signal the brain of satiety. However, sometimes, leptin resistance may inhibit this signal to the brain. This leads to constant hunger and overeating. Scientists have found that increased SIRT1 levels in laboratory mice prevent age-associated weight gain and increased leptin sensitivity. Improving SIRT1 genes through NAD+ intermediates (crucial for SIRT1 activation) may help control excessive hunger by sensitizing the body to leptin.

5. Preserves Lean Muscle: Activated SIRT1 genes help preserve lean muscle mass while burning fat. Sirtuins (proteins produced by the SIRT1 genes) increase skeletal muscle mass. The activated SIRT1 genes boost muscle growth and recovery. Therefore, age-associated muscle loss and exercise-induced muscle loss can be prevented.

6. Reduces Inflammation: Constant state of low-grade inflammation can cause cells to function abnormally. This leads to fat accumulation and obesity-related comorbidities (like diabetes and heart disease). Activated SIRT1 genes help reduce inflammation and reduce the risk of heart disease, tumors, and Alzheimer's disease. Now that we know how well the Sirtfood diet can work for weight loss, let us discuss the foods that help activate the SIRT1 genes.

What Are "Sirtfoods"?

Sirtfoods are the foods that activate the SIRT1 genes. Sirtfoods are mainly plant-based foods that contain powerful phytonutrients (plant nutrients). These activate the sirtuin-activating biochemicals, which otherwise only get activated in response to stress like fasting or exercising. When you consume these Sirtfoods, your body mimics the stress response without you having to fast or exercise. Hence, you burn calories/fat without losing muscle mass, without fasting, and without doing vigorous exercises. In the following section, we will take a quick look at the foods you can eat on the Sirtfood diet.

Breakfast Recipes

1. Not Your Everyday Apples

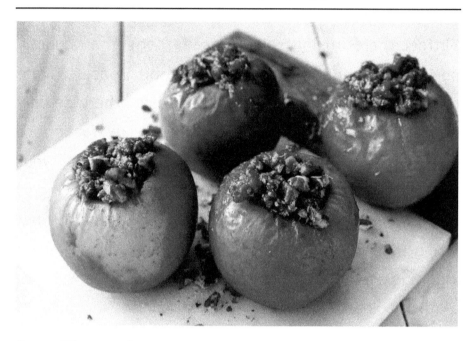

Prep Time: 10 minutes

Cooking Time: 20 minutes

Makes: 3 cups

Nutritional Facts

- ❖ Calories 130

- ❖ Total Fat 0g 0%

- ❖ Total Carbohydrate 34g 11%

- ❖ Cholesterol 0mg 0%

- ❖ Dietary Fiber 5g   20%

- ❖ Sodium 0mg   0%

- ❖ Sugars 25g

- ❖ Potassium 260mg   7%

- ❖ Protein   1g

- ❖ Vitamin A   2%

- ❖ Calcium 2%

- ❖ Vitamin C   8%

- ❖ Iron   2%

Calories from Fat 0 Percent Daily Values (%DV) are based on a 2,000 calorie diet.

Ingredients

- ❖ 3 medium apples (3" diameter)

- ❖ 1/2 cup raisins

- ❖ 2 teaspoons soft butter or margarine

- ❖ 2 teaspoons brown sugar

- ❖ 1/4 teaspoon cinnamon

Directions

- ❖ Preheat oven to 400 degrees.

- ❖ Wash the apples and chop them into small pieces.

- ❖ Mix apples with raisins, butter or margarine, sugar, and cinnamon.

- ❖ Place the mixture in a baking dish and cover loosely with foil. Bake for about 20 minutes.

- ❖ Cool slightly and enjoy!

- ❖ Refrigerate leftovers within 2 hours.

Notes

- ❖ Try serving this recipe with vanilla yogurt!

---

2. Oven French Toast

Prep Time: 10 minutes

Cooking Time: 30 minutes

Makes: 12 slices

Nutritional Facts

- ❖ Nutrition Facts
- ❖ Calories 580
- ❖ Calories from Fat 216
- ❖ % Daily Value
- ❖ Fat 24g37%
- ❖ Saturated Fat 13g81%
- ❖ Cholesterol 220mg73%
- ❖ Sodium 563mg24%
- ❖ Potassium 256mg7%
- ❖ Carbohydrates 74g25%
- ❖ Fiber 1g4%

- ❖ Sugar 37g 41%
- ❖ Protein 15g 30%
- ❖ Vitamin A 910IU 18%
- ❖ Vitamin C 0.1mg 0%
- ❖ Calcium 146mg 15%
- ❖ Iron 3.3mg 18%

Percent Daily Values are based on a 2000 calorie diet.

Ingredients

- ❖ 12 slices whole-grain bread
- ❖ 4 eggs or 8 egg whites
- ❖ 1 cup nonfat or 1% milk
- ❖ 1/4 cup packed brown sugar
- ❖ 1 teaspoon vanilla
- ❖ powdered sugar (optional)

Directions

- ❖ Preheat oven to 325 degrees.
- ❖ Lightly spray a cookie sheet with sides or two 9x13 inch pans with cooking spray.
- ❖ Lay the slices of bread flat on the pan with the sides touching.
- ❖ Beat egg, milk, brown sugar, and vanilla until very well blended.
- ❖ Pour mixture over bread. Turn each slice over to ensure both sides are wet.

- ❖ Cover and refrigerate overnight or bake immediately for 30 minutes.

- ❖ Serve hot. Sprinkle lightly with powdered sugar (optional). Top with applesauce, fresh fruit, or yogurt.

Notes

- ❖ Serve with applesauce or yogurt.

- ❖ Add your favorite berries to the top for some color and a yummy taste!

---

3. Overnight Oatmeal

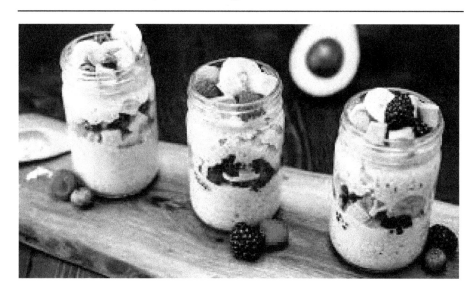

Prep Time: 15 minutes

Cooking Time: 6 hours

Makes: 4 cups

Nutritional Fact

- ❖ Calories: 236kcal,

- ❖ Carbohydrates: 34.5g,
- ❖ Protein: 6g, Fat: 10g,
- ❖ Saturated Fat: 0.5g,
- ❖ Sodium: 95mg,
- ❖ Fiber: 8.5g,
- ❖ Sugar: 11.5g

Ingredients

- ❖ 1 cup uncooked old fashioned rolled oats
- ❖ 1 cup low-fat yogurt
- ❖ 1/2 cup nonfat or 1% milk
- ❖ 1/2 cup berries, fresh or frozen
- ❖ 1/2 cup chopped apple (about 1/3 a medium apple [3" diameter])

Directions

- ❖ In a medium bowl, mix oats, yogurt, and milk.
- ❖ Add the fruit now or add just before eating.
- ❖ Cover and refrigerate the oatmeal mixture for 6-12 hours.
- ❖ For grab-and-go breakfasts, place scoops of the mixture in small dishes or spoon into small containers with lids.
- ❖ Refrigerate leftovers within 2 hours.

Notes

- ❖ Try other fresh, frozen, or canned fruits.

4. Overnight Oats For One

Prep Time: 5 minutes

Cooking Time: 6-12 hours

Makes: 1 cup

Nutrition Facts

* ❖ Calories: 389
* ❖ Water: 8%
* ❖ Protein: 16.9 grams
* ❖ Carbs: 66.3 grams
* ❖ Sugar: 0 grams
* ❖ Fiber: 10.6 grams
* ❖ Fat: 6.9 grams

Ingredients

* ❖ 1/3 cup old-fashioned oats
* ❖ 1/3 cup yogurt
* ❖ 1/3 cup milk
* ❖ 2 Tablespoons dry milk
* ❖ 1 dash cinnamon
* ❖ 1/2 cup bite-sized fruit (fresh, frozen, or canned)

Directions

* ❖ In a small bowl or 12-ounce mug, mix oats, yogurt, milk, dry milk, and cinnamon or other spice.

❖ Add 1/2 cup bite-size fruit now or add just before serving.

❖ Cover and refrigerate the oatmeal mixture for 6 to 12 hours.

Notes

❖ You can make this a higher calorie meal by using whole milk dairy products. You can use alternative milk or yogurt such as soy, almond, or oat in place of dairy products but the nutrients will be different.

5. Rice Salad

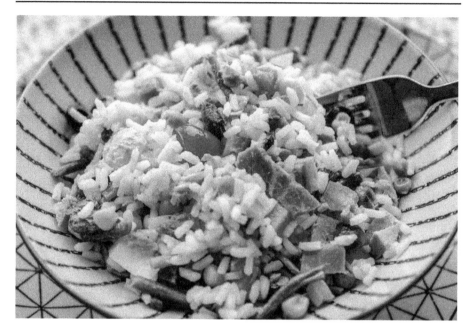

Prep Time: 10 minutes

Makes: 4 cups

Nutritional Facts

❖ Calories: 140

❖ Total Fat: 2g

❖ Sodium: 180mg

❖ Carbohydrates: 28g

❖ Sugars: 11g

❖ Protein: 3g

❖ Dietary Fiber: 3g

Ingredients

- ❖ 2 cups cooked rice, cooled
- ❖ ¼ cup chopped celery
- ❖ 1 apple, chopped (about 1 ½ cups)
- ❖ ¼ cup raisins
- ❖ 2 tablespoons chopped almonds
- ❖ ½ cup low-fat plain yogurt
- ❖ 2 teaspoons orange juice
- ❖ 2 teaspoons sugar

Instructions

- ❖ Combine rice, celery, apple, raisins, and almonds in a medium bowl and mix well.
- ❖ Combine yogurt, orange juice, and sugar and stir until sugar dissolves.
- ❖ Pour the yogurt mixture over the rice mixture and mix well. Cover and refrigerate until ready to serve.
- ❖ Refrigerate leftovers within 2 hours.

Notes

- ❖ Add any of your favorite fruits for variety.
- ❖ Make this a whole grain recipe by using brown rice instead of white rice.

6. Peach Sundae

Prep Time: 10 minutes

Cooking Time: 5 minutes

Makes: 5 cups

Nutritional Facts

❖ Calories 237

❖ Calories from Fat 63 (26.6%)

❖ % Daily Value

❖ Total Fat 7g

❖ Saturated fat 4.2g

❖ Trans fat 0.3g

❖ Cholesterol 21mg

❖ Sodium 98mg 5%

❖ Carbohydrates 37.6g

❖ Net carbs 37.6g

❖ Sugar 32.7g

❖ Fiber 0g 0%

❖ Protein 5.6g

❖ Vitamins and minerals

❖ Calcium 174.1mg   18%

❖ Fatty acids

❖ Amino acids

The Percent Daily Values are based on a 2,000 calorie diet, so your values may change depending on your calorie needs.

Ingredients

❖ 1 Tablespoon margarine or butter

❖ 2 cups chopped or sliced peaches (frozen, canned, and drained, or about 3-4 medium fresh)

❖ 3 Tablespoons packed brown sugar

❖ 1/4 teaspoon ground cinnamon

❖ 3 cups (24 ounces) low-fat yogurt (try peach, vanilla, or raspberry)

Directions

❖ Melt margarine in a medium skillet over medium heat (300 degrees in an electric skillet).

❖ Add peaches, brown sugar, and cinnamon. Stir occasionally until peaches are hot. Remove from heat.

❖ Spoon yogurt into five individual bowls. Top with warm peaches.

❖ Refrigerate leftovers within 2 hours.

Notes

❖ For a little crunch, sprinkle with granola, graham cracker, or gingersnap cookie crumbs.

Lunch Recipes

7. Fiesta Barley Salad

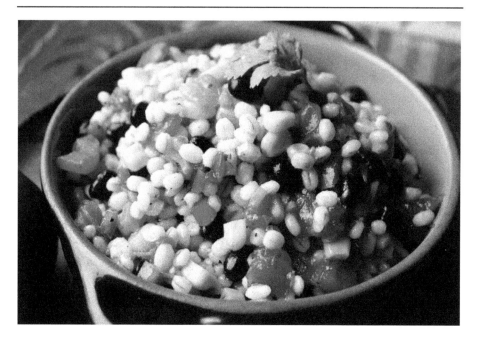

Prep Time: 15 minutes

Cooking Time: 45 minutes

Makes: 7 cups

Nutritional Facts

❖ Calories:310.8

❖ Protein: 23g

❖ Carbohydrates: 42.2g

❖ Exchange Other Carbs: 3

- ❖ Dietary Fiber: 10.5g
- ❖ Sugars: 7.4g
- ❖ Fat: 6.4g
- ❖ Saturated Fat: 1.1g
- ❖ Cholesterol: 35.9mg
- ❖ Vitamin A Iu: 2263.6IU
- ❖ Niacin Equivalents: 9.3mg
- ❖ Vitamin B6: 0.4mg
- ❖ Vitamin C: 19mg
- ❖ Folate: 93.6mcg
- ❖ Calcium: 95.1mg
- ❖ Iron: 3.8mg
- ❖ Magnesium: 40mg
- ❖ Potassium: 540mg
- ❖ Sodium: 1605.9mg
- ❖ Thiamin: 0.1mg
- ❖ Calories From Fat: 57.5
- ❖ Percent Of Calories From Carbs: 53
- ❖ Percent Of Calories From Fat: 18
- ❖ Percent Of Calories From Protein: 28
- ❖ Percent Of Calories From Sat Fat: 3

Percent Daily Values are based on a 2,000 calorie diet. Your daily values may be higher or lower depending on your calorie needs.

Ingredients

❖ 1 cup dry barley

❖ 3 cups of water

❖ 1/4 cup raisins, or other dried fruit

❖ 1 cup frozen peas, or other vegetables (fresh, frozen, or canned and drained)

❖ 3 cups lettuce, washed and chopped

❖ 1 can (15 ounces) mandarin oranges, drained

❖ 1/2 cup green onions, sliced thin (can use any onions)

❖ 1 Tablespoon vinegar (rice vinegar or any others)

❖ 3 Tablespoons vegetable oil

Directions

❖ Place barley and water in a 2-3 quart saucepan. Bring to boil, then turn to low. Cover and cook for 45 minutes.

❖ Rinse cooked barley briefly in cold water. Drain.

❖ Add remaining ingredients. Mix well.

❖ Refrigerate leftovers within 2 hours.

Notes

❖ Try substituting different fruits and vegetables.

---

8. Fish Salad

Prep Time: 20 minutes

Cooking Time: 30 minutes

Makes: 6 cups

Nutritional Facts

❖ Calories: 280

❖ Fat: 12.5g

❖ Sodium: 86mg

❖ Carbohydrates: 0g

❖ Fiber: 0g

❖ Sugars: 0g

❖ Protein: 39.2g

Ingredients

❖ 2 pounds fish fillets (try cod, tilapia, snapper, or others)

❖ 1/4 teaspoon each salt and pepper

❖ 2 cups shredded cabbage or lettuce

❖ 2 cups chopped vegetables (try tomatoes, cucumber, carrots, corn, green onions, celery, avocado)

❖ 1/2 cup low-fat ranch dressing

* 1/2 cup salsa

Directions

* Season fish with salt and pepper. Cook by your favorite method until it appears opaque and flakes apart easily (see Notes).

* Mix cabbage or lettuce with other vegetables of your choice. Add chunks of fish. Drizzle with ranch dressing and salsa.

* Refrigerate leftovers within 2 hours.

Cook Fish:

In A Skillet - Spray Or Lightly Oil A Skillet.

* Add seasoned fish and cook over medium heat (300 degrees in an electric skillet) until the flesh starts to appear white.

* Turn fish over and cook until it flakes easily.

* In the Oven - Put seasoned fish in a baking pan and cover with foil. Bake in a 350-degree oven until fish flakes.

* Under a Broiler - Place seasoned fish on a broiler pan.

* Broil several inches from the heat until the fish is opaque throughout and flakes easily.

* To make tacos instead of salad: Warm tortillas. Layer cabbage or lettuce, vegetables of your choice, and fish on the tortilla. Drizzle with ranch dressing and salsa. Fold in half.

9. Fish Tacos

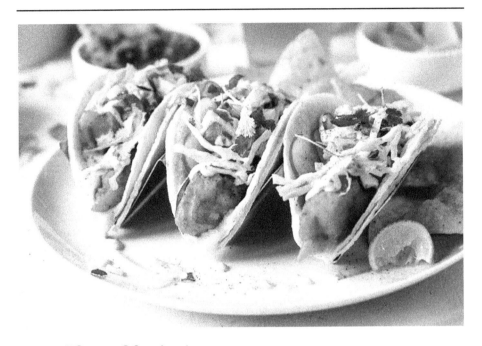

Prep Time: 20 minutes

Cooking Time: 20 minutes

Makes: 8 tacos

Nutritional Facts

- ❖ Calories: 200
- ❖ Calories From Fat: 25
- ❖ Total Fat: 2.5g
- ❖ Sodium: 250mg
- ❖ Carbohydrates: 21g
- ❖ Sugars: 5g
- ❖ Protein: 23g

❖ Dietary Fiber: 2g

Ingredients

Fish

❖ 2 pounds cod fillets

❖ 3 Tablespoons lime juice (about 2 limes)

❖ 1 tomato, chopped

❖ 1/2 onion, chopped

❖ 3 Tablespoons cilantro, chopped

❖ 1 teaspoon oil

❖ 1/4 teaspoon cayenne pepper (optional)

❖ 1/4 teaspoon black pepper

❖ 1/4 teaspoon salt

Slaw

❖ 2 cups shredded red cabbage

❖ 1/2 cup green onions, chopped

❖ 3/4 cup nonfat sour cream

❖ 3/4 cup salsa

❖ 8 corn tortillas (6-inch)

Directions

❖ Preheat oven to 350 degrees.

❖ Place fish in a baking dish.

❖ Mix lime juice, tomato, onion, cilantro, oil, peppers, and salt and spoon on top of fillets.

- ❖ Cover loosely with aluminum foil to keep fish moist.

- ❖ Bake 15-20 minutes or until fish flakes.

- ❖ Mix cabbage and onion; mix sour cream and salsa and add to cabbage mixture.

- ❖ Divide cooked fish among tortillas. Add 1/4 cup of slaw to each. Fold over and enjoy!

- ❖ Refrigerate leftovers within 2 hours.

Notes

- ❖ Freeze extra lime juice to use later.

10. Fried Rice With Pork

Prep Time: 15 minutes

Cooking Time: 15-20 minutes

Makes: 4 cups

Nutritional Facts

- ❖ Calories: 260

- ❖ Calories From Fat: 90

- ❖ Total Fat: 10g

- ❖ Sodium: 310mg

- ❖ Carbohydrates: 26g

- ❖ Sugars: 1g

- ❖ Protein: 14g

- ❖ Dietary Fiber: 1g

Ingredients

- ❖ 2 Tablespoons low-sodium soy sauce
- ❖ 1/2 teaspoon garlic powder
- ❖ 1 teaspoon black pepper
- ❖ 1/2 pound lean pork, ground or small cubes
- ❖ 1 teaspoon oil
- ❖ 1/4 cup carrot, sliced or grated
- ❖ 1 cup onion, chopped
- ❖ 1 cup chopped vegetables, fresh, frozen, or leftovers (try broccoli, celery, bell pepper, peas, or snow peas)
- ❖ 2 cups cooled, cooked rice, white or brown

Directions

- ❖ Mix soy sauce, garlic powder, and pepper in a small dish. Set aside.
- ❖ In a large skillet over medium-high heat, sauté pork in oil until just lightly browned. If using ground pork, break into crumbles as it cooks.
- ❖ Add carrots, onion, and chosen vegetables. Sauté until tender, stirring frequently.
- ❖ Stir in rice and seasoning mixture, breaking up any clumps of rice. Continue to heat and stir until heated through.
- ❖ Refrigerate leftovers within 2 hours.

Notes

❖ Leftover, cold rice makes a better texture than freshly cooked warm rice.

❖ Substitute 1 cup cooked or canned pork. Add with the vegetables.

❖ Mix ½ teaspoon sesame oil or some ginger powder with the soy sauce.

❖ Add sliced green onions or bite-sized pineapple (fresh, frozen, or canned).

11. Fruited Tabbouleh

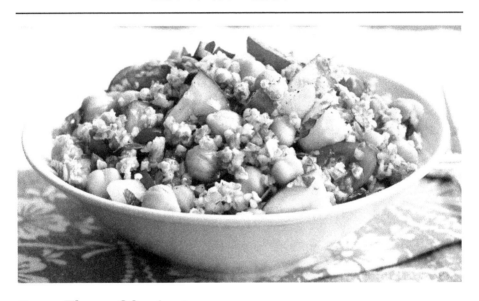

Prep Time: 30 minutes

Cooking Time: 5 minutes

Chill Time: 30 minutes

Makes: 4 cups

Nutritional Facts

❖ 160 to 170 calories

- ❖ 37 to 29 grams carbohydrates

- ❖ 2 to 3 grams protein

- ❖ 0 to 1 grams fat

- ❖ 1 to 2 grams fiber

- ❖ 1.7 milligrams iron (10 percent DV)

Ingredients

- ❖ 1 1/2 cups broth, chicken or vegetable

- ❖ 1 cup bulgur wheat

- ❖ 1 cup grapes, cut in half or quarters

- ❖ 1/3 cup minced onion

- ❖ 3 Tablespoons chopped fresh mint leaves or parsley

- ❖ 1 small orange, peeled and diced or 3/4 cup (one 11-ounce can) mandarin oranges, drained

Dressing

- ❖ 2 Tablespoons oil

- ❖ 2 Tablespoons lemon juice or vinegar

- ❖ 2 teaspoons sugar

- ❖ 1/4 teaspoon salt

- ❖ 1/2 teaspoon ground ginger

- ❖ 1/2 teaspoon ground cumin

- ❖ 1 teaspoon black pepper

Directions

❖ Heat broth to boiling, stir in bulgur and turn off the heat. Cover and set aside for 25 minutes.

❖ Remove the cover and fluff the bulgur with a fork. Let cool at least 5 minutes.

❖ Stir in grapes, onion, mint or parsley, and orange.

❖ In a small bowl or jar with a tight lid, mix or shake together the dressing ingredients. Pour over bulgur mixture and toss well. Chill until ready to serve.

❖ Refrigerate leftovers within 2 hours.

12. Garden Sloppy Joes

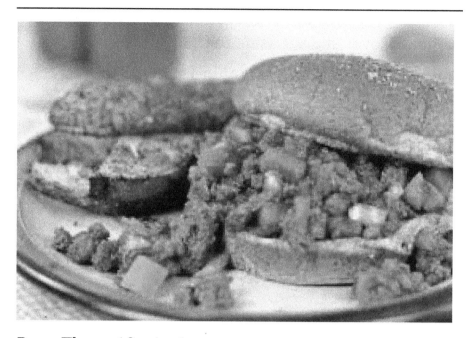

Prep Time: 10 minutes

Cooking Time: 20 minutes

Makes: 6 sandwiches

Nutritional Facts

- ❖ Calories: 140
- ❖ Calories From Fat: 25
- ❖ Total Fat: 2.5g
- ❖ Sodium: 230mg
- ❖ Carbohydrates: 19g
- ❖ Sugars: 6g
- ❖ Protein: 10g

❖ Dietary Fiber: 3g

Ingredients

❖ 1 onion, chopped

❖ 1 carrot, chopped or shredded

❖ 1 green pepper, chopped

❖ 1 pound lean ground meat (15% fat) (turkey, chicken, or beef)

❖ 1 can (8 ounces) tomato sauce

❖ 1 can (15 ounces) whole tomatoes, crushed

❖ 1 can (8 ounces) mushrooms or 1/2 pound chopped fresh mushrooms

❖ 1/4 cup barbecue sauce

❖ 6 whole wheat buns, split in half to make 12

Directions

❖ Saute onions, carrots, green pepper, and ground meat in a 2-3 quart saucepan over medium-high heat for 5 minutes.

❖ Add tomato sauce, crushed tomatoes, mushrooms, and barbecue sauce.

❖ Bring to a boil. Reduce heat and simmer for 15 to 20 minutes or until thick, stirring occasionally.

❖ Toast buns if desired. Spoon sauce over bun halves. Serve open-faced.

❖ Refrigerate leftovers within 2 hours.

Notes

❖ Add your favorite fresh, canned, or frozen chopped vegetables.

Try whole-wheat English muffins instead of buns.

Dinner Recipes

13. Garden Vegetable Cakes

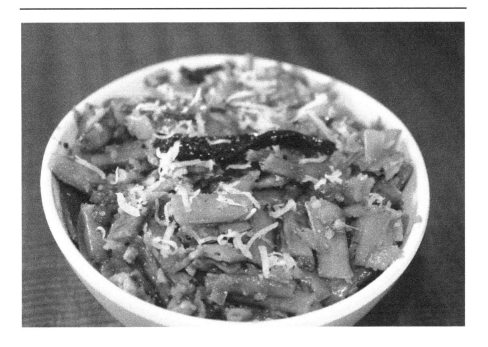

Prep Time: 20 minutes

Cooking Time: 15 minutes

Makes: 8 cakes

Nutritional Facts

- ❖ Calories: 150
- ❖ Total Fat: 6g
- ❖ Sodium: 370mg
- ❖ Carbohydrates: 15g

- ❖ Sugars: 2g
- ❖ Protein: 9g
- ❖ Dietary Fiber: 1g

Ingredients

- ❖ 1/4 cup grated Parmesan cheese
- ❖ 1/3 cup all-purpose flour
- ❖ 1/2 teaspoon baking powder
- ❖ 1/4 teaspoon dill weed
- ❖ 1/4 teaspoon each salt and pepper
- ❖ 4 eggs (or 1 cup egg substitute)
- ❖ 2 Tablespoons minced green onion with tops
- ❖ 2 teaspoons lemon juice
- ❖ 1 clove garlic or 1/4 teaspoon garlic powder
- ❖ 1 1/2 cups shredded vegetables (unpeeled zucchini (drained and pressed), potato, carrots, bell pepper, celery, sweet potato, or yam)

Directions

- ❖ In a medium bowl, stir together cheese, flour, baking powder, dill weed, salt, and pepper.
- ❖ Beat in eggs, green onions, lemon juice, and garlic until well blended. Stir all shredded vegetables into the batter.

- ❖ Heat skillet or griddle over medium-high heat (350 degrees in an electric skillet). Lightly spray or foil with cooking spray. For each vegetable cake, pour 1/3 cup batter onto a hot skillet or griddle. Cook on both sides until golden brown. Serve warm.
- ❖ Refrigerate leftovers within 2 hours.

Notes

- ❖ Top with low-fat sour cream and tomato slices.
- ❖ Precook "harder" vegetables like carrots and potatoes, if desired.

14. Garlic Ginger Ramen With Beef

Prep Time: 10 minutes

Cooking Time: 15 minutes

Makes: 6 cups

Nutritional Facts

- ❖ Calories: 150
- ❖ Calories From Fat 80
- ❖ Total Fat: 8g
- ❖ Sodium: 380mg
- ❖ Carbohydrates: 23g

- Sugars: 2g
- Protein: 11g
- Dietary Fiber: 2g

Ingredients

- 1/2 pound lean ground beef (15% fat)
- 2 cups of water
- 2 packages oriental flavor instant ramen-style noodles, broken into small pieces
- 16 ounces frozen Asian-style vegetables, or any other frozen vegetables
- 2 green onions, thinly sliced
- 1 Tablespoon fresh ginger or 1/4 teaspoon ground ginger
- 2 cloves garlic, minced, or 1/2 teaspoon garlic powder

Directions

- In a large skillet over medium-high heat (350 degrees F in an electric skillet), brown ground beef and cook until no longer pink. Drain fat.
- Add 2 cups of water and ONE seasoning packet to cooked beef and mix well.
- Add frozen vegetables, green onion, ginger, and garlic and bring to a boil over high heat.

❖ Add ramen noodles, reduce heat to low, and simmer 3-5 minutes until vegetables are tender, stirring occasionally.

15. Ham And Vegetable Chowder

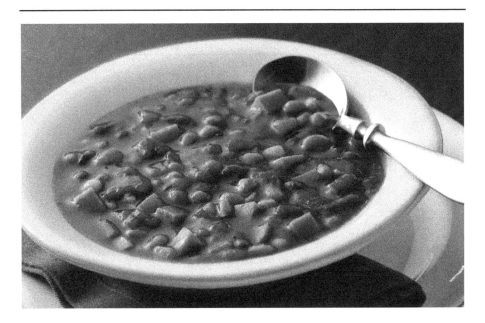

Prep Time: 15 minutes

Cooking Time: 20 minutes

Makes: 10 cups

Nutritional Facts

❖ Calories: 341.3
❖ Protein: 16.3g
❖ Carbohydrates: 16g

- ❖ Exchange Other Carbs: 1
- ❖ Dietary Fiber: 2.1g
- ❖ Sugars: 5.4g
- ❖ Fat: 23.9g
- ❖ Saturated Fat: 12.1g
- ❖ Cholesterol: 55.3mg
- ❖ Vitamin A Iu: 4459IU
- ❖ Niacin Equivalents: 4.3mg
- ❖ Vitamin B6: 0.2mg
- ❖ Vitamin C: 34.7mg
- ❖ Folate: 62mcg
- ❖ Calcium: 444mg
- ❖ Iron: 1.1mg
- ❖ Magnesium: 34.2mg
- ❖ Potassium: 374.7mg
- ❖ Sodium: 927.1mg
- ❖ Thiamin: 0.2mg
- ❖ Calories From Fat: 214.7

Ingredients

- ❖ 1 Tablespoon vegetable oil
- ❖ 1 small onion, chopped
- ❖ 1/2 head cabbage, chopped (about 6 cups)
- ❖ 1 large potato, peeled and diced

- ❖ 2 cans (14.5 ounces each) low-sodium chicken broth (see notes)
- ❖ 2 cans (15 ounces each) cream-style corn
- ❖ 1 cup chopped lean ham (8% fat)
- ❖ 1/2 teaspoon pepper
- ❖ 1/2 cup grated cheddar cheese

Directions

- ❖ Heat oil in 4 quarts (or larger) saucepan. Saute onion, cabbage, and potato over medium heat, stirring often, until soft, about 10 minutes.
- ❖ Add chicken broth, corn, ham, and pepper.
- ❖ Cover and simmer until potato is tender, about 10 minutes
- ❖ Serve hot, sprinkled with cheese.
- ❖ Refrigerate leftovers within 2 hours.

Notes

- ❖ Broth can be canned or made using bouillon. For each cup of broth use 1 cup very hot water and 1 teaspoon or 1 cube bouillon.
- ❖ Leave the skin on the potato for added fiber.
- ❖ For a vegetarian soup, substitute vegetable broth for the chicken broth and beans for the ham.

16. Kale And White Bean Soup

Prep Time: 15 minutes

Cooking Time: 15 minutes

Makes: 5 cups

Nutritional Facts

- ❖ Calories: 277.3
- ❖ Protein: 9.6g
- ❖ Carbohydrates: 50.9g
- ❖ Exchange Other Carbs: 3.5
- ❖ Dietary Fiber: 10.3g
- ❖ Sugars: 4.8g
- ❖ Fat: 4.5g
- ❖ Saturated Fat: 0.6g
- ❖ Vitamin A Iu: 9137.4IU
- ❖ Niacin Equivalents: 3.3mg
- ❖ Vitamin B6: 0.5mg
- ❖ Vitamin C: 106.1mg
- ❖ Folate: 52.7mcg
- ❖ Calcium: 171.3mg
- ❖ Iron: 5.1mg
- ❖ Magnesium: 60.8mg
- ❖ Potassium: 1041.7mg

❖ Sodium: 372.2mg

❖ Thiamin: 0.1mg

Ingredients

❖ 1 cup onion, chopped (1 medium onion)

❖ 4 cloves garlic, minced or 1 teaspoon garlic powder

❖ 1 Tablespoon butter or margarine

❖ 2 cups broth (chicken or vegetable)

❖ 1 1/2 cups cooked white beans (1 can - 15.5 ounces, drained and rinsed)

❖ 1 3/4 cups diced tomatoes (1 can - 14.5 ounces with juice)

❖ 1 tablespoon Italian seasoning

❖ 3 cups kale, chopped (fresh or frozen)

Directions

❖ In a saucepan over medium-high heat, sauté onion and garlic in butter or margarine until soft.

❖ Add broth, white beans, and tomatoes; stir to combine.

❖ Bring to a boil; reduce heat, cover, and simmer for about 5 minutes.

❖ Add the kale and Italian seasoning. Simmer until kale has softened, 3 to 5 minutes. Serve warm.

- ❖ Refrigerate leftovers within 2 hours.

Notes

- ❖ 1 bunch fresh kale (about 8 cups, chopped)

---

17. Leek And Mushroom Orzo

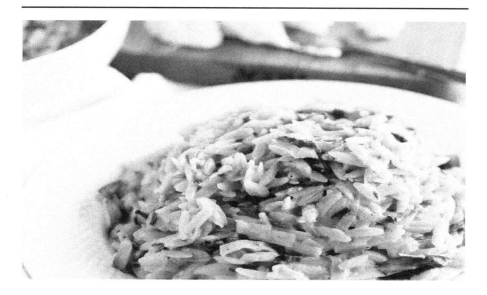

Prep Time: 15 minutes

Cooking Time: 30 minutes

Makes: 4 cups

Nutritional Facts

- ❖ Calories 150
- ❖ Total Fat 4g
- ❖ Saturated Fat 1.5g

- ❖ Trans Fat 0g
- ❖ Cholesterol 5mg
- ❖ Sodium 300mg
- ❖ Total Carbohydrate 24g
- ❖ Dietary Fiber 2g
- ❖ Total Sugars 3g
- ❖ Protein 5g

Ingredients

- ❖ 2 cups leeks, chopped
- ❖ 1 Tablespoon oil
- ❖ 2 cups mushrooms, sliced
- ❖ 1 cup dry orzo (rice-shaped pasta)
- ❖ 2 cups low-sodium chicken or vegetable broth
- ❖ 1 1/2 cups tomato, chopped
- ❖ 3 Tablespoons cream cheese
- ❖ 1 teaspoon garlic powder
- ❖ 1/4 teaspoon each salt and pepper

Directions

- ❖ Sauté leeks in oil in a medium skillet over medium heat, stirring occasionally, until the leeks are soft (about 5 minutes).
- ❖ Add mushrooms and cook until soft (about 5 minutes).

- ❖ Stir in the orzo and toast lightly, stirring frequently, for about 3 minutes.
- ❖ Add broth and bring to a boil. Reduce heat to simmer, stirring occasionally, until the orzo is almost tender, about 8 minutes.
- ❖ Add the tomatoes and simmer until orzo is tender (about 2 minutes).
- ❖ Remove from heat and stir in cream cheese, garlic powder, salt, and pepper. Serve warm.

18. Lentil Confetti Salad

Prep Time: 15 minutes

Cooking Time: 20 minutes

Makes: 4 cups

Nutritional Facts

- ❖ Calories: 102kcal
- ❖ Carbohydrates: 20g
- ❖ Protein: 7g
- ❖ Fat: 3g
- ❖ Sodium: 255mg
- ❖ Fiber: 9g
- ❖ Sugar: 1g

Ingredients

- ❖ 1/2 cup dry lentils
- ❖ 1 1/2 cups water
- ❖ 1/4 teaspoon salt
- ❖ 1 cup cooked brown rice
- ❖ 1/2 cup Italian dressing
- ❖ 1/2 cup tomatoes, seeded and diced
- ❖ 1/4 cup green peppers, seeded and chopped (about 1/2 a small pepper)
- ❖ 3 Tablespoons chopped onion
- ❖ 2 Tablespoons chopped celery
- ❖ 6 sliced pimento-stuffed green olives
- ❖ 2 teaspoons chopped fresh parsley (optional)

Directions

- ❖ Wash and drain lentils. Place in a saucepan, add water and salt.
- ❖ Bring to boil, reduce heat, and simmer, covered about 20 minutes. Do not overcook. The lentils should be tender with skin intact. Drain immediately.
- ❖ Combine the lentils with cooked rice, pour dressing over mixture, and refrigerate until cool.
- ❖ Add rest of the ingredients, except parsley, mix well.
- ❖ Garnish with parsley before serving (optional).

Snack Recipes

19. Fruit Salad

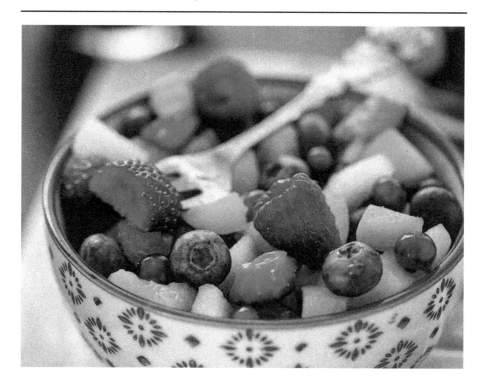

Prep Time: 10 minutes

Makes: 5 cups

Nutritional Facts

- ❖ Calories: 50
- ❖ Calories From Fat: 5
- ❖ Total Fat: 0g
- ❖ Sodium: 15mg

- ❖ Carbohydrates: 12g
- ❖ Sugars: 10g
- ❖ Protein: 1g
- ❖ Dietary Fiber: 1g
- ❖ Cholesterol: 0mg

Ingredients

- ❖ 2 cups strawberries
- ❖ 1 cup blueberries
- ❖ 1 cup grapes
- ❖ 1 can (8 ounces) pineapple chunks
- ❖ 6 ounces nonfat lemon yogurt

Directions

- ❖ Drain juice from pineapple. Cut grapes and strawberries into halves.
- ❖ Combine strawberries, blueberries, grapes, and pineapple chunks in a large bowl.
- ❖ Drizzle yogurt over fruit. Toss lightly to coat.
- ❖ Refrigerate leftovers within 2 hours.

20. Glass of Sunshine Flavored Water

Prep Time: 5 minutes

Chill Time: 2 hours

Makes: 8 cups

Ingredients

- ❖ 1 orange
- ❖ 2 quarts water

Directions

- ❖ Scrub the orange thoroughly under cool running water.
- ❖ Slice the orange into thin slices, with or without the peel.
- ❖ Combine the orange slices and water in a pitcher and refrigerate for 2 hours before serving.
- ❖ Drink within 2 days for best quality.

Notes

- ❖ Keep It Safe! Do not mix batches of flavored water. Use it up, clean the container, then make a fresh batch.

21. Healthy Carrot Cake Cookies

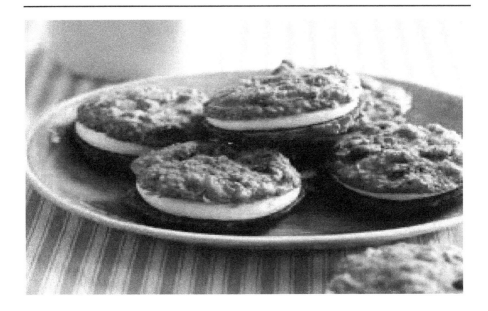

Prep Time: 20 minutes

Cooking Time: 15 minutes

Makes: 48 cookies

Nutritional Facts

❖ Calories: 170

❖ Calories From Fat: 50

❖ Total Fat: 6g

❖ Sodium: 105mg

❖ Carbohydrates: 15g

❖ Sugars: 14g

❖ Protein: 3g

- ❖ Dietary Fiber: 2g
- ❖ Cholesterol: 15mg

Ingredients

- ❖ 1/2 cup packed brown sugar
- ❖ 1/2 cup sugar
- ❖ 1/2 cup oil
- ❖ 1/2 cup applesauce or fruit puree
- ❖ 2 eggs
- ❖ 1 teaspoon vanilla
- ❖ 1 cup flour
- ❖ 1 cup whole wheat flour
- ❖ 1 teaspoon baking soda
- ❖ 1 teaspoon baking powder
- ❖ 1/4 teaspoon salt
- ❖ 1 teaspoon ground cinnamon
- ❖ 1/2 teaspoon ground nutmeg
- ❖ 1/2 teaspoon ground ginger
- ❖ 2 cups old fashioned rolled oats (raw)
- ❖ 1 1/2 cups finely grated carrots (about 3 large carrots)
- ❖ 1 cup raisins or golden raisins

Directions

- ❖ Heat oven to 350 degrees.

- In a large bowl, mix sugars, oil, applesauce, eggs, and vanilla thoroughly.
- In a separate bowl, stir dry ingredients together.
- Blend dry ingredients into the wet mixture. Stir in raisins and carrots.
- Drop by teaspoonfuls on a greased baking sheet.
- Bake 12 to 15 minutes until golden brown.
- Store in an airtight container.

---

22.   Kale Dip

Prep Time: 10 minutes

Cooking Time: 5 minutes

Makes: 1½ cups

Nutritional Facts

- Calories: 30
- Calories From Fat: 10
- Total Fat: 1g
- Sodium: 105mg
- Carbohydrates: 2g
- Sugars: 1g
- Protein: 3g
- Dietary Fiber: 0g

❖ Cholesterol: 0mg

Ingredients

❖ 1 1/2 teaspoons oil
❖ 1 clove garlic, minced or 1/4 teaspoon garlic powder
❖ 3 cups kale, thinly sliced
❖ 1/8 teaspoon salt
❖ 1 cup low-fat cottage cheese
❖ 1/2 teaspoon red pepper flakes or 1/4 teaspoon cayenne pepper
❖ 1 Tablespoon lemon juice

Directions

❖ Heat oil in a pan over medium heat. Add garlic and kale and season with salt. Cook, uncovered, stirring occasionally until tender, about 3 to 4 minutes. Let cool.
❖ Transfer kale to a blender. Add cottage cheese and puree until smooth.
❖ Season with red pepper flakes and lemon juice.
❖ Refrigerate leftovers within 2 hours.

Notes

❖ 1 bunch fresh kale (about 8 cups, chopped)

- ❖ No blender? Make a chunky version! Finely chop kale and garlic before cooking. Mash dip with a fork.
- ❖ Try adding onion or garlic powder, dill weed, or curry powder for a flavor boost.
- ❖ Can be made ahead and refrigerated for up to 3 days.
- ❖ Serve with fresh vegetables or Food Hero Baked Tortilla Chips.
- ❖ Freeze extra lemon juice to use later.

23. Lemony Garbanzo Bean Dip

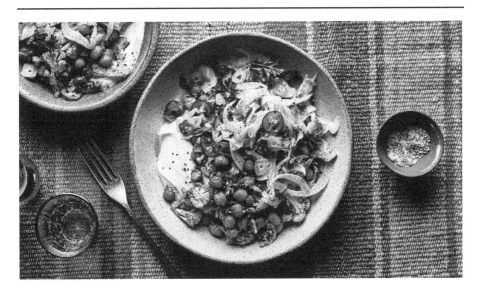

Prep Time: 5 minutes

Makes: 2 cups

Nutritional Facts

- ❖ Calories: 40
- ❖ Calories From Fat: 20
- ❖ Total Fat: 2g
- ❖ Sodium: 45mg
- ❖ Carbohydrates: 4g
- ❖ Sugars: 1g
- ❖ Protein: 3g
- ❖ Dietary Fiber: 0g
- ❖ Cholesterol: 5mg

Ingredients

- ❖ 1 can (15 ounces) garbanzo beans, drained and rinsed
- ❖ 1/2 cup low-fat sour cream
- ❖ 2 Tablespoons lemon juice
- ❖ 1 Tablespoon oil
- ❖ 1/2 teaspoon cumin
- ❖ 1 teaspoon hot sauce
- ❖ 2 cloves garlic, minced or 1/2 teaspoon garlic powder
- ❖ 2 Tablespoons or more cilantro, chopped

Directions

- ❖ For a smooth dip, place all ingredients in a blender and blend until smooth. OR for a chunky dip, mash beans well with a fork or potato masher then stir in remaining ingredients.

❖ Add additional liquid as needed for desired consistency.

❖ Refrigerate leftovers within 2 hours.

Notes

❖ Serve with fresh vegetables or Food Hero Baked Tortilla Chips.

❖ Freeze extra lemon juice to use later.

❖ Cook your dry beans. One can (15 ounces) is about 1 1/2 to 1 3/4 cups drained beans.

---

24. Low-Fat Pumpkin Bread

Prep Time: 15 minutes

Cooking Time: 1 hour

Makes: 20 slices

Nutritional Facts

❖ Calories: 120

❖ Calories From Fat: 5

❖ Total Fat: 1g

❖ Sodium: 45mg

- ❖ Carbohydrates: 25g
- ❖ Sugars: 17g
- ❖ Protein: 2g
- ❖ Dietary Fiber: 1g
- ❖ Cholesterol: 25mg

Ingredients

- ❖ Non-stick cooking spray or oil
- ❖ 1 1/2 cups whole wheat flour
- ❖ 1 1/3 cups all-purpose flour
- ❖ 2 teaspoons baking powder
- ❖ 1 teaspoon baking soda
- ❖ 1/2 teaspoon salt
- ❖ 1 teaspoon cinnamon
- ❖ 1/2 teaspoon ground cloves
- ❖ 1/4 teaspoon ground ginger
- ❖ 1/4 teaspoon nutmeg
- ❖ 4 eggs
- ❖ 1 cup canned pumpkin
- ❖ 1 cup applesauce
- ❖ 3/4 cup packed brown sugar
- ❖ 3/4 cup sugar

Directions

❖ Preheat oven to 350 degrees. Lightly coat an 8 ½ x 4 ½ -inch loaf pan with cooking spray or oil and set aside.

❖ In a medium bowl, combine flours, baking powder, baking soda, cinnamon, salt, cloves, ginger, and nutmeg.

❖ In a separate bowl, combine the eggs, pumpkin, applesauce, brown sugar, and sugar. Mix until well combined.

❖ Add the wet ingredients to the dry ingredients. Stir only until the dry ingredients become moistened. Be careful not to over mix.

❖ Pour batter into loaf pan and spread into the corners.

❖ Bake for about 60 minutes or until a wooden pick inserted into the center of the loaf comes out clean.

❖ Remove from the oven and let cool in the pan for 10 minutes.

❖ Remove from pan and let cool completely on a rack. Slice to serve.

❖ Wrap in plastic or foil to store for several days or freeze for up to a month.

Dessert Recipes

25.   Ginger Almond Asparagus

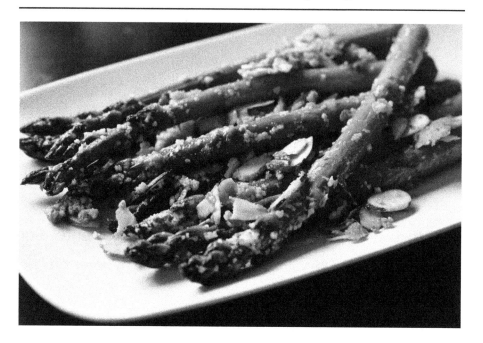

Prep Time: 5 minutes

Cooking Time: 10 minutes

Makes: 3 cups

Nutritional Facts

❖ Calories: 60

❖ Calories From Fat: 35

❖ Total Fat: 4g

❖ Sodium: 150mg

- ❖ Carbohydrates: 5g
- ❖ Sugars: 2g
- ❖ Protein: 3g
- ❖ Dietary Fiber: 2g
- ❖ Cholesterol: 0mg

Ingredients

- ❖ ¾ pound asparagus, washed and trimmed (2 1/2 cups sliced)
- ❖ 1 teaspoon oil
- ❖ 3 tablespoons slivered almonds
- ❖ ¼ teaspoon salt
- ❖ Pinch of black pepper
- ❖ ¼ teaspoon sugar
- ❖ ⅛ teaspoon ginger powder

Instructions

- ❖ Slice the asparagus diagonally into pieces about ¾ inch long.
- ❖ Heat oil in a large skillet over medium heat. Add remaining ingredients. Stir and sauté until asparagus is a brighter green, 3-5 minutes.
- ❖ Reduce heat to medium-low; cover and cook until the asparagus is just fork-tender. Avoid overcooking.

Shake the pan occasionally to prevent sticking or burning.

❖ Refrigerate leftovers within 2 hours.

---

26.   Pumpkin Breakfast Cookies

Prep Time: 20 minutes

Cooking Time: 10 to 12 minutes per baking sheet

Makes: 48 cookies

Nutritional Facts

❖ Calories: 200
❖ Calories From Fat: 70
❖ Total Fat: 8g
❖ Sodium: 110mg
❖ Carbohydrates: 31g
❖ Sugars: 2g
❖ Protein: 19g
❖ Dietary Fiber: 2g
❖ Cholesterol: 15mg

Ingredients

❖ 1 can (15 ounces) pumpkin (1 3/4 cup)
❖ 1 cup packed brown sugar

- ❖ 2 eggs
- ❖ 1/2 cup vegetable oil
- ❖ 1 1/2 cups all-purpose flour
- ❖ 1 1/4 cups whole-wheat flour
- ❖ 1 Tablespoon baking powder
- ❖ 2 teaspoons cinnamon
- ❖ 1 teaspoon nutmeg
- ❖ 1/4 teaspoon ground ginger
- ❖ 1/2 teaspoon salt
- ❖ 1 cup raisins or other dried fruit
- ❖ 1 cup chopped nuts, any type

Directions

- ❖ Preheat oven to 400 degrees F.
- ❖ In a large bowl, stir together the pumpkin, brown sugar, eggs, and oil. Mix well until smooth.
- ❖ In a separate bowl, stir the flours, baking powder, cinnamon, nutmeg, ground ginger, and salt together. Add to the pumpkin mixture and mix well.
- ❖ Stir in the raisins and nuts.
- ❖ Drop the dough by a tablespoon onto a greased baking sheet, 1 inch apart.
- ❖ Gently flatten each cookie with the back of a spoon.

❖ Bake 10-12 minutes until the tops are dry and begin to brown.

Notes

❖ Refrigerate or freeze leftover cookies in a sealed container. They will remain fresh for 3 to 4 days in the refrigerator or 4 to 6 weeks in the freezer.

---

27. Pumpkin Fruit Dip

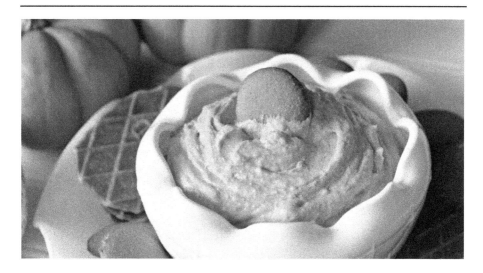

Prep Time: 5 minutes

Makes: 3 cups

Nutritional Facts

❖ Calories: 200
❖ Calories From Fat: 5

- ❖ Total Fat: 0.5g
- ❖ Sodium: 25mg
- ❖ Carbohydrates: 8g
- ❖ Sugars: 7g
- ❖ Protein: 1g
- ❖ Dietary Fiber: 1g
- ❖ Cholesterol: 5mg

Ingredients

- ❖ 1 can (15 ounces) pumpkin (about 1 ¾ cups cooked pumpkin)
- ❖ 1 cup low-fat ricotta cheese or plain yogurt or low-fat cream cheese
- ❖ 3/4 cup sugar
- ❖ 1 1/2 teaspoons cinnamon
- ❖ 1/2 teaspoon nutmeg

Directions

- ❖ In a large bowl, combine pumpkin, ricotta cheese or yogurt or cream cheese, cinnamon, and nutmeg. Add sugar a little at a time to reach the desired sweetness. Stir until smooth.

Notes

❖ Serve with apple slices, bananas, or grapes.

❖ Try using a mixture of ricotta, yogurt, or cream cheese.

❖ For a smoother texture, use a hand mixer or food processor to mix ingredients.

---

28.   Gingerbread Pancakes

Prep Time: 10 minutes

Cook Time: 5 minutes

Makes: 8 pancakes(4 inch)

Nutritional Facts

❖ Calories: 200

❖ Calories From Fat: 50

❖ Total Fat: 6g

❖ Sodium: 530mg

❖ Carbohydrates: 33g

❖ Sugars: 11g

❖ Protein: 7g

❖ Dietary Fiber: 2g

❖ Cholesterol: 45mg

Ingredients

- ½ cup whole wheat flour
- ½ cup all-purpose flour
- ½ teaspoon salt
- ½ teaspoon baking soda
- 2 teaspoons pumpkin pie spice
- 1 egg
- 2 tablespoons molasses
- 1 tablespoon vegetable oil
- 1 cup low-fat buttermilk

Instructions

- Mix dry ingredients in a bowl.
- In another bowl, beat egg. Stir in molasses, oil and buttermilk.
- Pour milk mixture into dry ingredients; stir together lightly.
- Lightly spray a large skillet or griddle with non-stick cooking spray or lightly wipe with oil. Heat skillet or griddle over medium-high heat (350 degrees in an electric skillet). For each pancake, pour about 1/4 cup of batter onto the hot griddle.
- Cook until pancakes are puffed and dry around edges. Turn and cook other side until golden brown.

❖ Refrigerate leftovers within 2 hours.

Notes

❖ No pumpkin pie spice? Use 1/2 teaspoon cinnamon, 1/2 teaspoon dry ginger, and 1/8 teaspoon cloves or nutmeg.

❖ No buttermilk? Place 1 Tablespoon of lemon juice or vinegar in measuring cup and fill to the 1 cup line with milk. Stir and let set to thicken slightly.

❖ To see if skillet is hot enough, sprinkle with a few drops of water. If drops skitter around, heat is just right.

❖ Top with applesauce, fresh fruit or yogurt.

29. Raspberry Fruit Dip

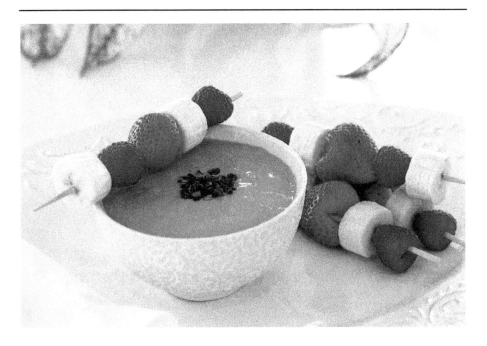

Prep Time: 5 minutes

Makes: 8 servings

Nutritional Facts

- ❖ Calories: 60
- ❖ Calories From Fat: 0
- ❖ Total Fat: 0g
- ❖ Sodium: 25mg
- ❖ Carbohydrates: 14g
- ❖ Sugars: 11g
- ❖ Protein: 2g

- ❖ Dietary Fiber: 2g
- ❖ Cholesterol: 0mg

Ingredients

- ❖ 1/2 cup raspberries fresh or frozen/thawed
- ❖ 1 Tablespoon sugar
- ❖ 1 cup plain nonfat or low-fat yogurt
- ❖ 3 pears or apples, sliced for serving

Directions

- ❖ In a small bowl, mash the raspberries with sugar. Stir in the yogurt.
- ❖ Serve with cut fruit.
- ❖ Refrigerate leftovers within two hours

30. Raspberry Oatmeal Bars

Prep Time: 20 minutes

Cooking Time: 45 minutes

Makes: 12 bars (2 inches x 2.5 inches)

Nutritional Facts

- ❖ Calories: 100
- ❖ Calories From Fat: 30
- ❖ Total Fat: 3.5g

- ❖ Sodium: 25mg
- ❖ Carbohydrates: 17g
- ❖ Sugars: 7g
- ❖ Protein: 2g
- ❖ Dietary Fiber: 2g
- ❖ Cholesterol: 10mg

Ingredients

1. Crust And Topping:

- ❖ 1/2 cup all-purpose flour
- ❖ 1/4 cup brown sugar
- ❖ 1 cup quick-cooking oats
- ❖ 3 Tablespoons margarine or butter
- ❖ 2 Tablespoons applesauce
- ❖ 1 Tablespoon orange juice

2. Filling:

- ❖ 1 Tablespoon all-purpose flour
- ❖ 1 Tablespoon brown sugar
- ❖ 1 1/2 teaspoons orange juice
- ❖ 2 cups raspberries (fresh or frozen)

Directions

❖ preheat oven to 375 degrees F. Spray or lightly oil an 8"x 8" baking pan.

❖ Crust and topping: Mix flour and sugar in a bowl. Cut margarine or butter into mixture until crumbly. Mix in oats. Set half aside for topping.

❖ To remaining mixture, stir in applesauce and orange juice. Press in the bottom of the baking pan.

❖ Filling: Combine flour, sugar, juice, and raspberries. Mix well.

❖ Spread filling on crust. Sprinkle with topping.

❖ Bake 40-45 minutes. Cool. Cut into 12 bars.

Drinks Recipes

31. Peach Yogurt Smoothie

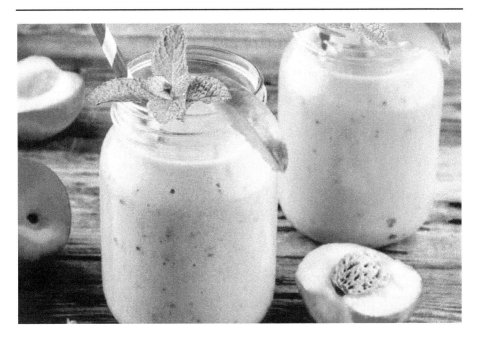

Prep Time: 10 minutes

Makes: 3 cups

Nutritional Facts

- ❖ Calories: 130
- ❖ Total Fat: 1g
- ❖ Sodium: 160mg
- ❖ Carbohydrates: 23g
- ❖ Sugars: 20g

- ❖ Protein: 8g
- ❖ Dietary Fiber: 1g

Ingredients

- ❖ 1 cup low-fat yogurt (try peach, vanilla, or lemon)
- ❖ 1/3 cup nonfat dry milk
- ❖ 1/2 banana
- ❖ 3/4 cup orange juice
- ❖ 1/2 cup frozen peaches

Directions

- ❖ Put all ingredients into a blender.
- ❖ Blend until smooth.
- ❖ Refrigerate leftovers within 2 hours.

Notes

- ❖ 1 cup chopped or sliced peaches (about 1.5 to 2 medium fresh)
- ❖ Serve as a snack or dessert during the summer months.

32.   Peanut Power Smoothie

Prep Time: 10 minutes

Makes: 4 cups

Nutritional Facts

❖ Calories: 180
❖ Total Fat: 8g
❖ Sodium: 115mg
❖ Carbohydrates: 22g
❖ Sugars: 13g
❖ Protein: 7g
❖ Dietary Fiber: 3g

Ingredients

❖ 1/4 cup peanut butter
❖ 1 3/4 cups banana (or any other fresh or canned and drained fruit)
❖ 1/4 cup nonfat dry milk powder
❖ 1 1/2 cups cold water

Directions

❖ Put all ingredients in the blender. Blend on low until smooth, and serve.

❖ Refrigerate leftovers within 2 hours.

Notes

❖ To avoid peanuts or peanut butter, try sunflower seeds or sunflower seed butter.

---

33.   Popeye Power Smoothie

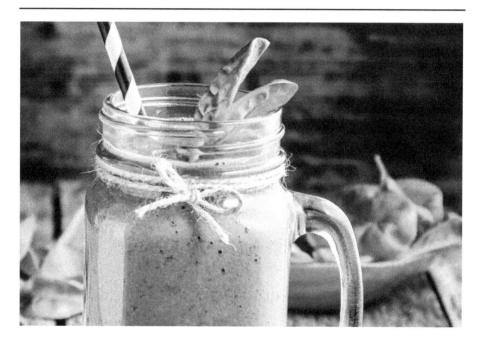

Prep Time: 10 minutes

Makes: 4 cups

Nutritional Facts

❖ Calories: 90

❖ Total Fat: 0.5g

- ❖ Sodium: 35mg
- ❖ Carbohydrates: 20g
- ❖ Sugars: 15g
- ❖ Protein: 3g
- ❖ Calcium: 77mg
- ❖ Vitamin D: 0mcg
- ❖ Vitamin A: 81mcg
- ❖ Vitamin C: 42mg
- ❖ Iron: 1mg
- ❖ Potassium: 355mg

Ingredients

- ❖ 1 cup of orange juice
- ❖ 1/2 cup pineapple juice
- ❖ 1/2 cup low-fat plain or vanilla yogurt
- ❖ 1 banana, peeled and sliced
- ❖ 2 cups fresh spinach leaves
- ❖ 2 cups crushed ice

Directions

- ❖ Combine all ingredients in a blender.
- ❖ Puree until completely smooth.
- ❖ Serve immediately.
- ❖ Refrigerate leftovers within 2 hours.

Notes

❖ For a thicker smoothie, use frozen fruit or vegetables instead of ice.

❖ Use any type of juice, even juice from canned pineapple.

---

34.   Pumpkin Smoothie In Cup

Prep Time: 5 minutes

Makes: 1 cup

Nutritional Facts

❖ Calories: 200

❖ Total Fat: 2.5g

❖ Sodium: 120mg

❖ Carbohydrates: 38g

❖ Sugars: 34g

❖ Protein: 9g

❖ Dietary Fiber: 9g

Ingredients

❖ 2/3 cup low-fat vanilla yogurt or 1 container (6 ounces)

❖ 1/4 cup canned pumpkin

- ❖ 2 teaspoons brown sugar
- ❖ 1/4 teaspoon cinnamon
- ❖ 1/8 teaspoon nutmeg (optional)

Directions

- ❖ Combine all ingredients in a bowl or blender.
- ❖ Mix until smooth and serve.
- ❖ Refrigerate leftovers within 2 hours.

Notes

- ❖ Top with granola or nugget type cereal for extra crunch.
- ❖ Extra canned pumpkin can be frozen to use later in main dishes, soups, chili, or baked goods.
- ❖ Tastes great as a dip with cut fruit or graham crackers.

35. Tropical Smoothie

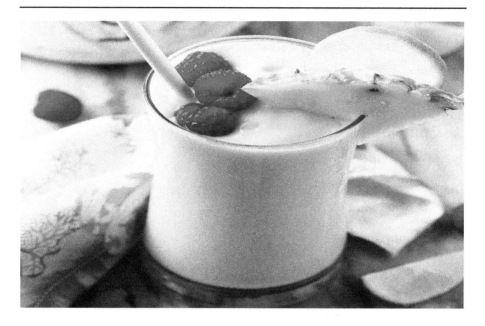

Prep Time: 5 minutes

Makes: 5 cups

Nutritional Facts

* Calories: 140
* Total Fat: 1g
* Sodium: 45mg
* Carbohydrates: 32g
* Sugars: 26g
* Protein: 4g
* Dietary Fiber: 3g

Ingredients

- ❖ 1 cup nonfat or 1% milk
- ❖ 2 cups pineapple chunks (fresh, frozen, or canned and drained)
- ❖ 1 banana
- ❖ 1 cup of cold water

Directions

- ❖ Put all ingredients in a blender. Put the lid on tightly.
- ❖ Blend until smooth.
- ❖ Pour into cups or glasses. Serve chilled.
- ❖ Refrigerate or freeze extra portions for a fast, healthy snack.

Notes

- ❖ For a thicker smoothie, use frozen fruit instead of fresh fruit.

36.   Un-beet-able Berry Smoothie

Prep Time: 5 minutes

Makes: 4 cups

Nutritional Facts

❖ Calories: 110

❖ Total Fat: 0g

❖ Sodium: 70mg

❖ Carbohydrates: 26g

❖ Sugars: 16g

❖ Protein: 2g

❖ Calcium: 93mg

❖ Vitamin D: 1mcg

❖ Vitamin A: 40mcg

❖ Vitamin C: 20mg

❖ Iron: 1mg

❖ Potassium: 266mg

Ingredients

❖ 1 cup pineapple juice

❖ 1 cup low-fat plain or vanilla yogurt

❖ 1 1/2 cups fresh or frozen berries, any type

❖ 1/2 cup beets, canned or cooked

❖ 1 small frozen banana (optional)

Directions

❖ Combine all ingredients in a blender.

❖ Blend until smooth.

❖ Serve immediately.

❖ Refrigerate or freeze leftovers within 2 hours.

Notes

❖ For a thicker smoothie, use frozen fruit instead of fresh fruit.

❖ Try adding 1/2 teaspoon vanilla if you use plain yogurt.

The Best Sirtfood Recipes

37. **Turmeric Chicken & Kale Salad with Honey Lime Dressing-Sirt Food Recipes**

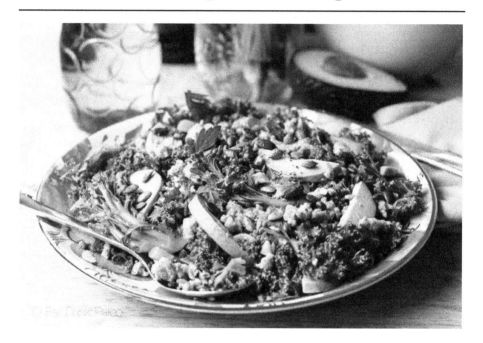

Prep Time: 20 mins

Cook Time: 10 mins

Total Time: 30 mins

Notes: If preparing ahead of time, dress the salad 10 minutes before serving. Chicken can be replaced with beef mince, chopped prawns, or fish. Vegetarians could use chopped mushrooms or cooked quinoa.

Serves: 2

Ingredients

1. For The Chicken

* 1 teaspoon ghee or 1 tbsp coconut oil
* ½ medium brown onion, diced
* 250-300 g / 9 oz. chicken mince or diced up chicken thighs
* 1 large garlic clove, finely diced
* 1 teaspoon turmeric powder
* 1teaspoon lime zest
* Juice of ½ lime
* ½ teaspoon salt + pepper

2. For The Salad

* 6 broccolini stalks or 2 cups of broccoli florets
* 2 tablespoons pumpkin seeds (pepitas)
* 3 large kale leaves, stems removed and chopped
* ½ avocado, sliced
* Handful of fresh coriander leaves, chopped
* Handful of fresh parsley leaves, chopped

For The Dressing

* 3 tablespoons lime juice

- ❖ 1 small garlic clove, finely diced or grated
- ❖ 3 tablespoons extra-virgin olive oil (I used 1 tablespoon avocado oil and * 2 tablespoons EVO)
- ❖ 1 teaspoon raw honey
- ❖ ½ teaspoon wholegrain or Dijon mustard
- ❖ ½ teaspoon sea salt and pepper

Instructions

1. Heat the ghee or coconut oil in a small frying pan over medium-high heat. Add the onion and sauté on medium heat for 4-5 minutes, until golden. Add the chicken mince and garlic and stir for 2-3 minutes over medium-high heat, breaking it apart.

2. Add the turmeric, lime zest, lime juice, salt, and pepper and cook, stirring frequently, for a further 3-4 minutes. Set the cooked mince aside.

3. While the chicken is cooking, bring a small saucepan of water to boil. Add the broccolini and cook for 2 minutes. Rinse under cold water and cut into 3-4 pieces each.

4. Add the pumpkin seeds to the frying pan from the chicken and toast over medium heat for 2 minutes,

stirring frequently to prevent burning. Season with a little salt. Set aside. Raw pumpkin seeds are also fine to use.

5. Place chopped kale in a salad bowl and pour over the dressing. Using your hands, toss and massage the kale with the dressing. This will soften the kale, kind of like what citrus juice does to fish or beef carpaccio – it 'cooks' it slightly.

6. Finally toss through the cooked chicken, broccolini, fresh herbs, pumpkin seeds, and avocado slices.

---

38.   Buckwheat Noodles With Chicken Kale & Miso Dressing-Sirt Food Recipes

---

Prep Time: 15 mins

Cook Time: 15 mins

Total Time: 30 mins

Serves: 2

Ingredients

For The Noodles

❖ 2-3 handfuls of kale leaves (removed from the stem and roughly cut)

- ❖ 150 g / 5 oz buckwheat noodles (100% buckwheat, no wheat)
- ❖ 3-4 shiitake mushrooms, sliced
- ❖ 1 teaspoon coconut oil or ghee
- ❖ 1 brown onion, finely diced
- ❖ 1 medium free-range chicken breast, sliced or diced
- ❖ 1 long red chili, thinly sliced (seeds in or out depending on how hot you like it)
- ❖ 2 large garlic cloves, finely diced
- ❖ 2-3 tablespoons Tamari sauce (gluten-free soy sauce)

For The Miso Dressing

- ❖ 1½ tablespoon fresh organic miso
- ❖ 1 tablespoon Tamari sauce
- ❖ 1 tablespoon extra-virgin olive oil
- ❖ 1 tablespoon lemon or lime juice
- ❖ 1 teaspoon sesame oil (optional)

Instructions

1. Bring a medium saucepan of water to boil. Add the kale and cook for 1 minute, until slightly wilted. Remove and set aside but reserve the water and bring it back to the boil. Add the soba noodles and cook according to the

package instructions (usually about 5 minutes). Rinse under cold water and set aside.

2. In the meantime, pan fry the shiitake mushrooms in a little ghee or coconut oil (about a teaspoon) for 2-3 minutes, until lightly browned on each side. Sprinkle with sea salt and set aside.

3. In the same frying pan, heat more coconut oil or ghee over medium-high heat. Sauté onion and chili for 2-3 minutes and then add the chicken pieces. Cook 5 minutes over medium heat, stirring a couple of times, then add the garlic, tamari sauce, and a little splash of water. Cook for a further 2-3 minutes, stirring frequently until chicken is cooked through.

4. Finally, add the kale and soba noodles and toss through the chicken to warm up.

5.Mix the miso dressing and drizzle over the noodles right at the end of cooking, this way you will keep all those beneficial probiotics in the miso alive and active.

39. Asian King Prawn Stir-Fry With Buckwheat Noodles – Sirt Food Recipes

Serves: 1

Ingredients:

- ❖ 150g shelled raw king prawns, deveined
- ❖ 2 tsp tamari (you can use soy sauce if you are not avoiding gluten)
- ❖ 2 tsp extra virgin olive oil
- ❖ 75g soba (buckwheat noodles)
- ❖ 1 garlic clove, finely chopped
- ❖ 1 bird's eye chili, finely chopped
- ❖ 1 tsp finely chopped fresh ginger
- ❖ 20g red onions, sliced
- ❖ 40g celery, trimmed and sliced
- ❖ 75g green beans, chopped
- ❖ 50g kale, roughly chopped
- ❖ 100ml chicken stock
- ❖ 5g lovage or celery leaves

Instructions:

1. Heat a frying pan over high heat, then cook the prawns in 1 teaspoon of the tamari and 1 teaspoon of the oil for 2–3 minutes. Transfer the prawns to a plate. Wipe the

pan out with kitchen paper, as you're going to use it again.

2. Cook the noodles in boiling water for 5–8 minutes or as directed on the packet. Drain and set aside.

Meanwhile, fry the garlic, chili and ginger, red onion, celery, beans, and kale in the remaining oil over medium-high heat for 2–3 minutes. Add the stock and bring to the boil, then simmer for a minute or two, until the vegetables are cooked but still crunchy.

3. Add the prawns, noodles, and lovage/celery leaves to the pan, bring back to the boil then remove from the heat and serve.

40. Baked Salmon Salad With Creamy Mint Dressing-Sirt Food Recipes

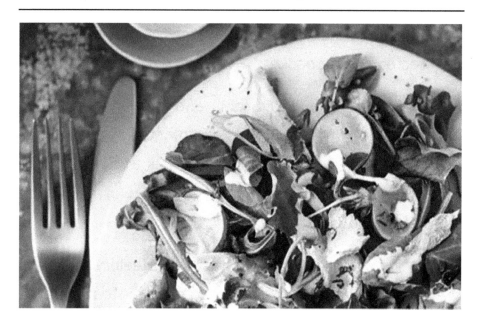

340 calories • 3 of your SIRT 5 a day

Baking the salmon in the oven makes this salad so simple.

Serves 1 • Ready in 20 minutes

Ingredients:

❖ 1 salmon fillet (130g)

❖ 40g mixed salad leaves

❖ 40g young spinach leaves

❖ 2 radishes, trimmed and thinly sliced

- ❖ 5cm piece (50g) cucumber, cut into chunks
- ❖ 2 spring onions, trimmed and sliced
- ❖ 1 small handful (10g) parsley, roughly chopped

For The Dressing:

- ❖ 1 tsp low-fat mayonnaise
- ❖ 1 tbsp natural yogurt
- ❖ 1 tbsp rice vinegar
- ❖ 2 leaves mint, finely chopped
- ❖ Salt and freshly ground black pepper

Instructions

1. Preheat the oven to 200°C (180°C fan/Gas 6).

2. Place the salmon fillet on a baking tray and bake for 16–18 minutes until just cooked through. Remove from the oven and set aside. The salmon is equally nice hot or cold in the salad. If your salmon has skin, simply cook skin side down and remove the salmon from the skin using a fish slice after cooking. It should slide off easily when cooked.

3. In a small bowl, mix the mayonnaise, yogurt, rice wine vinegar, mint leaves, and salt and pepper and leave to stand for at least 5 minutes to allow the

flavors to develop.

4. Arrange the salad leaves and spinach on a serving plate and top with the radishes, cucumber, spring onions, and parsley. Flake the cooked salmon onto the salad and drizzle the dressing over.

41. Fragrant Asian Hotpot-Sirt Food Recipes

185 calories

1 1/2 of you SIRT 5 a day

Serves 2 • Ready in 15 minutes

Ingredients

- ❖ 1 tsp tomato purée
- ❖ 1-star anise, crushed (or 1/4 tsp ground anise)
- ❖ Small handful (10g) parsley, stalks finely chopped
- ❖ Small handful (10g) coriander, stalks finely chopped
- ❖ Juice of 1/2 lime
- ❖ 500ml chicken stock, fresh or made with 1 cube
- ❖ 1/2 carrot, peeled and cut into matchsticks
- ❖ 50g broccoli, cut into small florets
- ❖ 50g beansprouts
- ❖ 100g raw tiger prawns
- ❖ 100g firm tofu, chopped

- ❖ 50g rice noodles, cooked according to packet instructions
- ❖ 50g cooked water chestnuts, drained
- ❖ 20g sushi ginger, chopped
- ❖ 1 tbsp good-quality miso paste

Instructions

1. Place the tomato purée, star anise, parsley stalks, coriander stalks, lime juice, and chicken stock in a large pan and bring to a simmer for 10 minutes.

2. Add the carrot, broccoli, prawns, tofu, noodles, and water chestnuts and simmer gently until the prawns are cooked through. Remove from the heat and stir in the sushi ginger and miso paste.

3. Serve sprinkled with the parsley and coriander leaves.

42. Lamb, Butternut Squash, And Date Tagine-Sirt Food Recipes

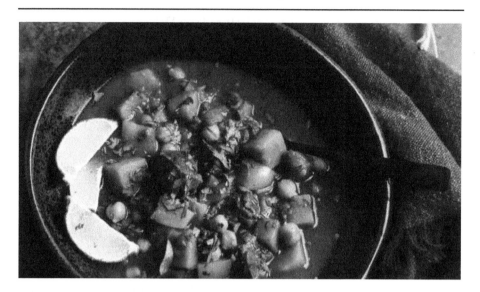

Prep Time: 15 mins

Cook Time: 1 hour 15 mins

Total Time: 1 hour 30 mins

Incredible warming Moroccan spices make this healthy tagine perfect for chilly autumn and winter evenings. Serve with buckwheat for an extra health kick!

Serves: 4

Ingredients

❖ 2 tablespoons olive oil

- ❖ 1 red onion, sliced
- ❖ 2cm ginger, grated
- ❖ 3 garlic cloves, grated or crushed
- ❖ 1 teaspoon chili flakes (or to taste)
- ❖ 2 teaspoons cumin seeds
- ❖ 1 cinnamon stick
- ❖ 2 teaspoons ground turmeric
- ❖ 800g lamb neck fillet, cut into 2cm chunks
- ❖ ½ teaspoon salt
- ❖ 100g Medjool dates, pitted and chopped
- ❖ 400g tin chopped tomatoes, plus half a can of water
- ❖ 500g butternut squash, chopped into 1cm cubes
- ❖ 400g tin chickpeas, drained
- ❖ 2 tablespoons fresh coriander (plus extra for garnish)
- ❖ Buckwheat, couscous, flatbreads, or rice to serve

Method

1.Preheat your oven to 140C.

2.Drizzle about 2 tablespoons of olive oil into a large ovenproof saucepan or cast iron casserole dish. Add the sliced onion and cook on a gentle heat, with the lid on, for about 5 minutes, until the onions are softened but not brown.

3.Add the grated garlic and ginger, chili, cumin, cinnamon, and turmeric. Stir well and cook for 1 more minute with the lid off. Add a splash of water if it gets too dry.

4.Next add in the lamb chunks. Stir well to coat the meat in the onions and spices and then add the salt, chopped dates, and tomatoes, plus about half a can of water (100-200ml).

5.Bring the tagine to the boil and then put the lid on and put in your preheated oven for 1 hour and 15 minutes.

6.Thirty minutes before the end of the cooking time, add in the chopped butternut squash and drained chickpeas. Stir everything together, put the lid back on and return to the oven for the final 30 minutes of cooking.

7.When the tagine is ready, remove from the oven and stir through the chopped coriander. Serve with buckwheat, couscous, flatbreads, or basmati rice.

Notes

If you don't own an ovenproof saucepan or cast iron casserole dish, simply cook the tagine in a regular saucepan up until it has to go in the oven and then transfer the tagine into a regular lidded casserole dish before placing in the oven. Add on an extra 5 minutes of cooking time to allow for the fact that the casserole dish will need extra time to heat up.

43. Prawn Arrabbiata-Sirt Food Recipes

Serves: 1

Preparation Time: 35 – 40 minutes

Cooking Time: 20 – 30 minutes

Ingredients

* ❖ 125-150 g Raw or cooked prawns (Ideally king prawns)
* ❖ 65 g Buckwheat pasta
* ❖ 1 tbsp Extra virgin olive oil
* ❖ For arrabbiata sauce
* ❖ 40 g Red onion, finely chopped
* ❖ 1 Garlic clove, finely chopped
* ❖ 30 g Celery, finely chopped
* ❖ 1 Bird's eye chili, finely chopped
* ❖ 1 tsp Dried mixed herbs
* ❖ 1 tsp Extra virgin olive oil
* ❖ 2 tbsp White wine (optional)

- ❖ 400 g Tinned chopped tomatoes
- ❖ 1 tbsp Chopped parsley

Method

1. Fry the onion, garlic, celery, and chili, and dried herbs in the oil over medium-low heat for 1–2 minutes. Turn the heat up to medium, add the wine, and cook for 1 minute. Add the tomatoes and leave the sauce to simmer over medium-low heat for 20–30 minutes, until it has a nice rich consistency. If you feel the sauce is getting too thick simply add a little water.

2. While the sauce is cooking bring a pan of water to a boil and cook the pasta according to the packet instructions. When cooked to your liking, drain, toss with the olive oil and keep in the pan until needed.

3. If you are using raw prawns add them to the sauce and cook for a further 3–4 minutes until they have turned pink and opaque, add the parsley and serve. If you are using cooked prawns add them with the parsley, bring the sauce to the boil and serve.

4. Add the cooked pasta to the sauce, mix thoroughly but gently and serve.

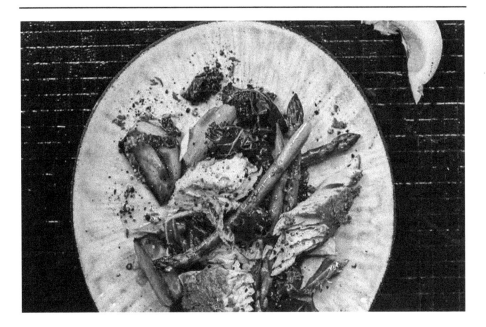

Serves: 1

Preparation Time: 10 – 15 minutes

Cooking Time: 10 minutes

Ingredients

- ❖ 125-150 g Skinned Salmon
- ❖ 1 tsp Extra virgin olive oil
- ❖ 1 tsp ground turmeric
- ❖ 1/4 Juice of a lemon
- ❖ For the spicy celery
- ❖ 1 tsp Extra virgin olive oil

- ❖ 40 g Red onion, finely chopped
- ❖ 60 g Tinned green lentils
- ❖ 1 Garlic clove, finely chopped
- ❖ 1 cm fresh ginger, finely chopped
- ❖ 1 Bird's eye chili, finely chopped
- ❖ 150 g Celery, cut into 2cm lengths
- ❖ 1 tsp Mild curry powder
- ❖ 130 g Tomato, cut into 8 wedges
- ❖ 100 ml Chicken or vegetable stock
- ❖ 1 tbsp Chopped parsley

Method

1. Heat the oven to 200C / gas mark 6.

2. Start with the spicy celery. Heat a frying pan over medium-low heat, add the olive oil, then the onion, garlic, ginger, chili, and celery. Fry gently for 2–3 minutes or until softened but not colored, then add the curry powder and cook for a further minute.

3. Add the tomatoes then the stock and lentils and simmer gently for 10 minutes. You may want to increase or decrease the cooking time depending on how crunchy you like your celery.

4. Meanwhile, mix the turmeric, oil, and lemon juice and rub over the salmon. Place on a baking tray and cook for 8–10 minutes.

5. To finish, stir the parsley through the celery and serve with the salmon.

---

45. Coronation Chicken Salad-Sirt Food Recipes

Serves: 1

Preparation Time: 5 minutes

Ingredients

- ❖ 75 g Natural yogurt
- ❖ Juice of 1/4 of a lemon
- ❖ 1 tsp Coriander, chopped
- ❖ 1 tsp ground turmeric
- ❖ 1/2 tsp Mild curry powder
- ❖ 100 g Cooked chicken breast, cut into bite-sized pieces
- ❖ 6 Walnut halves, finely chopped
- ❖ 1 Medjool date, finely chopped
- ❖ 20 g Red onion, diced
- ❖ 1 Bird's eye chili
- ❖ 40 g Rocket, to serve

Method

Mix the yogurt, lemon juice, coriander, and spices in a bowl. Add all the remaining ingredients and serve on a bed of the rocket.

---

46. Baked Potatoes With Spicy Chickpea Stew-Sirt Food Recipes

---

Prep Time: 10 mins

Cook Time: 1 hour

Serves: 4-6

Kind of Mexican Mole meets North African Tagine, this Spicy Chickpea Stew is unbelievably delicious and makes a great topping for baked potatoes, plus it just happens to be vegetarian, vegan, gluten-free, and dairy-free. And it contains chocolate.

Ingredients

- ❖ 4-6 baking potatoes, pricked all over
- ❖ 2 tablespoons olive oil
- ❖ 2 red onions, finely chopped
- ❖ 4 cloves garlic, grated or crushed
- ❖ 2cm ginger, grated

- ½ -2 teaspoons chili flakes (depending on how hot you like things)
- 2 tablespoons cumin seeds
- 2 tablespoons turmeric
- Splash of water
- 2 x 400g tins chopped tomatoes
- 2 tablespoons unsweetened cocoa powder (or cacao)
- 2 x 400g tins chickpeas (or kidney beans if you prefer) including the chickpea water DON'T DRAIN!!
- 2 yellow peppers (or whatever color you prefer!), chopped into bitesize pieces
- 2 tablespoons parsley plus extra for garnish
- Salt and pepper to taste (optional)
- Side salad (optional)

Method

1.Preheat the oven to 200C, meanwhile you can prepare all your ingredients.

2.When the oven is hot enough put your baking potatoes in the oven and cook for 1 hour or until they are done how you like them.

3.Once the potatoes are in the oven, place the olive oil and chopped red onion in a large wide saucepan and cook gently, with the lid on for 5 minutes, until the onions are soft but not brown.

4.Remove the lid and add the garlic, ginger, cumin, and chili. Cook for a further minute on low heat, then add the turmeric and a very small splash of water and cook for another minute, taking care not to let the pan get too dry.

5.Next, add in the tomatoes, cocoa powder (or cacao), chickpeas (including the chickpea water), and yellow pepper. Bring to the boil, then simmer on a low heat for 45 minutes until the sauce is thick and unctuous (but don't let it burn!). The stew should be done at roughly the same time as the potatoes.

6.Finally stir in the 2 tablespoons of parsley, and some salt and pepper if you wish, and serve the stew on top of the baked potatoes, perhaps with a simple side salad.

47. Kale And Red Onion Dhal With Buckwheat-Sirt Food Recipes

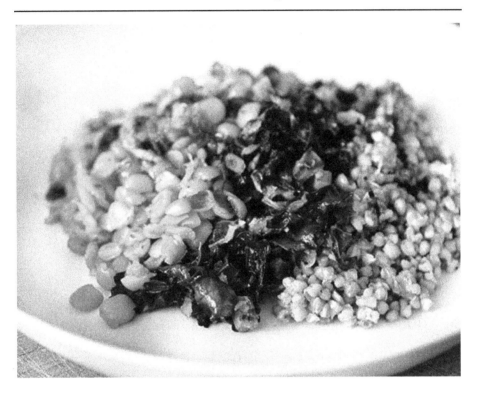

Prep Time: 5 mins

Cook Time: 25 mins

Total Time: 30 mins

Serves: 4

Delicious and very nutritious this Kale and Red Onion Dhal with Buckwheat are quick and easy to make and naturally gluten-free, dairy-free, vegetarian, and vegan.

Ingredients

- ❖ 1 tablespoon olive oil
- ❖ 1 small red onion, sliced
- ❖ 3 garlic cloves, grated or crushed
- ❖ 2 cm ginger, grated
- ❖ 1 birds eye chili, deseeded and finely chopped (more if you like things hot!)
- ❖ 2 teaspoons turmeric
- ❖ 2 teaspoons garam masala
- ❖ 160g red lentils
- ❖ 400ml coconut milk
- ❖ 200ml water
- ❖ 100g kale (or spinach would be a great alternative)
- ❖ 160g buckwheat (or brown rice)

Method

1.Put the olive oil in a large, deep saucepan and add the sliced onion. Cook on low heat, with the lid on for 5 minutes until softened.

2.Add the garlic, ginger, and chili and cook for 1 more minute.

3.Add the turmeric, garam masala, and a splash of water and cook for 1 more minute.

118

4.Add the red lentils, coconut milk, and 200ml water (do this simply by half filling the coconut milk can with water and tipping it into the saucepan).

5.Mix everything together thoroughly and cook for 20 minutes over a gentle heat with the lid on. Stir occasionally and add a little more water if the dhal starts to stick.

6.After 20 minutes add the kale, stir thoroughly and replace the lid, cook for a further 5 minutes (1-2 minutes if you use spinach instead!)

7.About 15 minutes before the curry is ready, place the buckwheat in a medium saucepan and add plenty of boiling water. Bring the water back to the boil and cook for 10 minutes (or a little longer if you prefer your buckwheat softer. Drain the buckwheat in a sieve and serve with the dhal.

48.   Chargrilled Beef With A Red Wine Jus, Onion Rings, Garlic Kale And Herb Roasted Potatoes-Sirt Food Recipes

Ingredients:

- ❖ 100g potatoes, peeled and cut into 2cm dice
- ❖ 1 tbsp extra virgin olive oil
- ❖ 5g parsley, finely chopped
- ❖ 50g red onion, sliced into rings
- ❖ 50g kale, sliced
- ❖ 1 garlic clove, finely chopped
- ❖ 120–150g x 3.5cm-thick beef fillet steak or 2cm-thick sirloin steak
- ❖ 40ml red wine
- ❖ 150ml beef stock
- ❖ 1 tsp tomato purée
- ❖ 1 tsp cornflour, dissolved in 1 tbsp water

Instructions:

1. Heat the oven to 220ºC/gas 7.

2. Place the potatoes in a saucepan of boiling water, bring back to the boil and cook for 4–5 minutes, then drain. Place in a roasting tin with 1 teaspoon of the oil and roast in the hot oven for 35–45 minutes. Turn the potatoes

every 10 minutes to ensure even cooking. When cooked, remove from the oven, sprinkle with the chopped parsley, and mix well.

3. Fry the onion in 1 teaspoon of the oil over medium heat for 5–7 minutes, until soft and nicely caramelized. Keep warm. Steam the kale for 2–3 minutes then drain. Fry the garlic gently in ½ teaspoon of oil for 1 minute, until soft but not colored. Add the kale and fry for a further 1–2 minutes, until tender. Keep warm.

4. Heat an ovenproof frying pan over high heat until smoking. Coat the meat in ½ a teaspoon of the oil and fry in the hot pan over medium-high heat according to how you like your meat done. If you like your meat medium it would be better to sear the meat and then transfer the pan to an oven set at 220°C/gas 7 and finish the cooking that way for the prescribed times.

5. Remove the meat from the pan and set aside to rest. Add the wine to the hot pan to bring up any meat residue. Bubble to reduce the wine by half, until syrupy and with a concentrated flavor.

6. Add the stock and tomato purée to the steak pan and bring to the boil, then add the cornflour paste to thicken

your sauce, adding it a little at a time until you have your desired consistency. Stir in any of the juices from the rested steak and serve with the roasted potatoes, kale, onion rings, and red wine sauce.

---

49.   Kale And Blackcurrant Smoothie-Sirt Food Recipes

---

86 calories 1 – 1/2 of your SIRT 5 a day

Serves 2 • Ready in 3 minutes

Ingredients

- ❖ 2 tsp honey
- ❖ 1 cup freshly made green tea
- ❖ 10 baby kale leaves, stalks removed
- ❖ 1 ripe banana
- ❖ 40 g blackcurrants, washed and stalks removed
- ❖ 6 ice cubes

Stir the honey into the warm green tea until dissolved. Whiz all the ingredients together in a blender until smooth. Serve immediately.

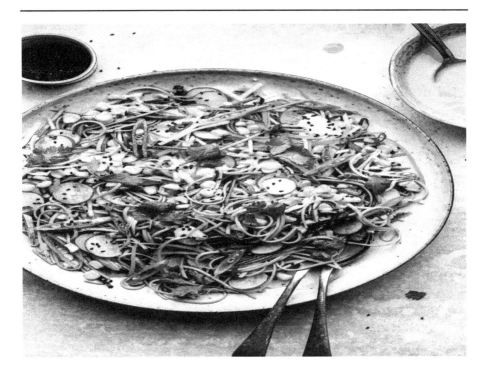

Serves: 1

Ingredients

- ❖ 50g buckwheat pasta(cooked according to the packet instructions) sirt food recipes
- ❖ large handful of rocket
- ❖ a small handful of basil leaves
- ❖ 8 cherry tomatoes, halved
- ❖ 1/2 avocado, diced
- ❖ 10 olives

* 1 tbsp extra virgin olive oil
* 20g pine nuts

Gently combine all the ingredients except the pine nuts and arrange on a plate or in a bowl, then scatter the pine nuts over the top.